Kids can cook: Fun recipes for young chefs

Chelsey Hoffman

Table of Contents

Introduction

- A warm welcome and an explanation of what the cookbook is about.
- Encourage kids to explore the world of cooking and discover the joy of creating delicious meals.

Section 1

Breakfast

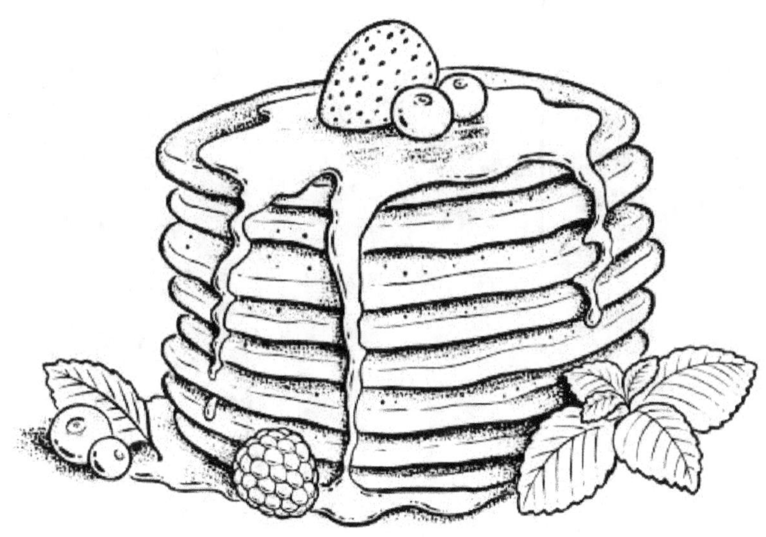

Pancake Pops

Serves: 24   Prep time: 10 min   Cook time: 23 min

INGREDIENTS

1 cup pancake mix

1/2 cup milk

1 egg

Maple syrup

Fruit chunks (e.g.,

strawberries, blueberries,

banana slices)

Wooden skewers

DIRECTIONS

1. In a mixing bowl, combine the pancake mix, milk, and egg. Mix until smooth.
2. Heat a non-stick pan over medium heat
3. Pour small circles of pancake batter onto the pan. Cook until bubbles form, then flip and cook the other side until golden brown
4. Let the pancakes cool slightly, then carefully slide them onto wooden skewers, alternating with fruit chunks
5. Serve with maple syrup for dipping. Enjoy your pancake pops!

Fruit Pizza

Serves: 12   Prep time: 20   Cook time: 20 min

INGREDIENTS

For the Sugar Cookie Crust:

1 1/2 cups all-purpose flour

1/2 cup powdered sugar

1/2 cup unsalted butter, softened

1 egg

1/2 teaspoon vanilla extract

1/4 teaspoon salt

For the Cream Cheese Topping:

8 ounces cream cheese, softened

1/2 cup granulated sugar

1 teaspoon vanilla extract

For the Fruit Topping:

A variety of fresh fruits such as

strawberries, kiwi, blueberries,

grapes, and pineapple

DIRECTIONS

1. Preheat your oven to 350°F (175°C)

2. In a mixing bowl, cream together the softened butter and powdered sugar until light and fluffy. Add the egg and vanilla extract, and mix until well combined

3. Gradually add the flour and salt to the mixture and mix until a soft dough forms

4. Press the cookie dough onto a pizza pan or a large baking sheet, forming a round or rectangular crust, about 1/4 inch thick

5. Bake the sugar cookie crust in the preheated oven for 12-15 minutes, or until it's lightly golden brown. Allow it to cool completely

6. While the crust is cooling, prepare the cream cheese topping. In a separate bowl, beat the softened cream cheese, granulated sugar, and vanilla extract until smooth and creamy

7. Once the cookie crust has cooled, spread the cream cheese topping evenly over the crust, leaving a small border around the edges

8. Arrange your choice of fresh fruits on top of the cream cheese layer. You can be creative with your fruit placement, making colorful patterns or designs

9. If desired, drizzle a little honey or warmed apricot preserves over the fruit for added sweetness and shine

10. Refrigerate the fruit pizza for at least an hour to let the flavors meld together and the cream cheese topping to set

11. Slice and serve your delicious fruit pizza, and enjoy!

Kids Breakfast Burritos

Serves: 8   Prep time: 35 min   Cook time: 35 min

INGREDIENTS

Flour tortillas

Eggs (2-4 per burrito, depending on your preference)

Breakfast meat (e.g., cooked sausage, bacon, or chorizo)

Vegetables (e.g., bell peppers, onions, and tomatoes)

Shredded cheese (cheddar, Monterey Jack, or your choice)

Salt and pepper to taste

Optional toppings: salsa, sour cream, guacamole

DIRECTIONS

1. Prepare your fillings
2. Cook
3. Place desire ingredients into tortillas and wrap

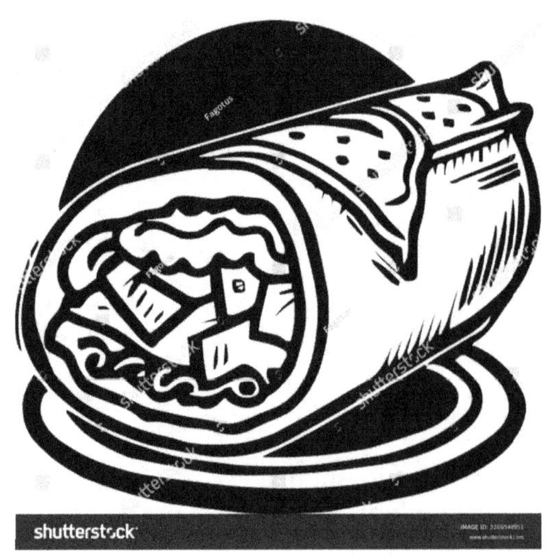

Section 2

Lunchtime Adventures

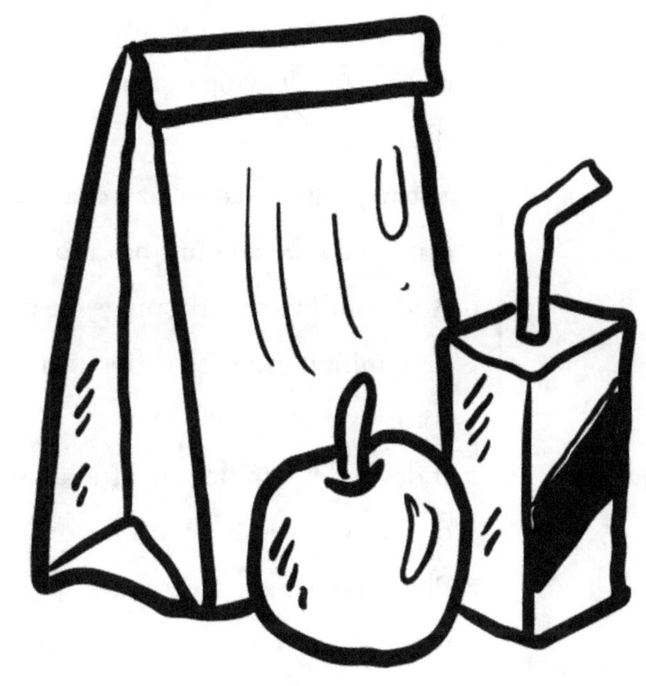

Mini Pizza

INGREDIENTS

Mini pizza crusts or small rounds of pizza dough

Pizza sauce

Shredded mozzarella cheese

Toppings of your choice

(e.g., pepperoni, sliced bell peppers, sliced onions, olives, mushrooms, cooked sausage, etc.)

Olive oil (for brushing)

Italian seasoning or dried oregano (optional)

DIRECTIONS

1. Preheat your oven to the temperature specified on the mini pizza crust packaging or around 425°F (220°C).
2. Place the mini pizza crusts or dough rounds on a baking sheet lined with parchment paper.
3. Brush a thin layer of olive oil over the surface of each mini pizza crust. This helps to prevent them from becoming too soggy from the sauce.
4. Spoon a generous amount of pizza sauce onto each mini pizza crust, leaving a small border around the edges for the crust.
5. Sprinkle shredded mozzarella cheese over the sauce. You can adjust the amount based on your preference.
6. Add your favorite toppings. Be creative and customize each mini pizza with different ingredients according to your taste.
7. If desired, sprinkle some Italian seasoning or dried oregano on top for extra flavor.
8. Place the baking sheet with the mini pizzas in the preheated oven.
9. Bake for 10-15 minutes or until the cheese is melted and bubbly, and the crust is golden brown.
10. Remove the mini pizzas from the oven, allow them to cool slightly, and then serve hot.

Veggie Wraps

Serves: 4   Prep time: 15 min   Cook time: 15 min

INGREDIENTS

Tortillas or flatbreads (whole wheat, spinach, or your preferred type)

Assorted fresh vegetables (e.g., lettuce, spinach, cucumber, bell peppers, carrots, red onion, avocado, tomato, etc.)

Hummus, tzatziki, or another preferred spread or sauce

Optional additions: olives, feta cheese, roasted red peppers, roasted chickpeas, or nuts for extra flavor and texture.

Seasonings and herbs (e.g., basil, cilantro, mint, or parsley)

DIRECTIONS

1. Prepare the vegetables: Wash and chop your choice of vegetables into thin strips or slices. You can mix and match vegetables based on your preferences and what you have on hand. The key is to have a variety of colors and textures for a satisfying wrap.

2. Heat the tortillas: You can warm the tortillas briefly in a dry skillet or microwave them for about 20 seconds until they are pliable. This step makes it easier to wrap the veggies.

3. Spread the sauce: Lay the warm tortilla flat and spread a generous layer of hummus, tzatziki, or your preferred spread/sauce across the center of the tortilla.

4. Add the vegetables: Arrange the chopped vegetables evenly over the spread, leaving some space around the edges to make folding and rolling the wrap easier.

5. Season and garnish: Sprinkle your choice of seasonings and herbs over the vegetables for added flavor. Fresh herbs like basil, cilantro, mint, or parsley work well. You can also add a pinch of salt and pepper if desired.

6. Optional extras: If you like, you can add olives, crumbled feta cheese, roasted red peppers, roasted chickpeas, or nuts to enhance the taste and texture of your veggie wrap.

7. Roll the wrap: Fold in the sides of the tortilla and then roll it up tightly from the bottom to enclose the filling. You can use a toothpick or wrap it in parchment paper to keep it together.

8. Serve and enjoy: Your veggie wrap is ready to eat! You can cut it in half diagonally for easier handling or enjoy it whole.

Grilled Cheese Sandwich

INGREDIENTS

2 slices of bread (common choices include white, whole wheat, or sourdough)

2-4 slices of cheese (common choices include cheddar, American, Swiss, or provolone)

Butter or margarine (for spreading)

Optional additions like bacon, tomatoes, onions, or herbs for flavor variation

DIRECTIONS

1. Heat a non-stick skillet or frying pan over medium-low heat.
2. Butter one side of each slice of bread. This will be the outside of the sandwich, and it helps give the bread a nice, crispy texture.
3. Place one slice of bread, buttered side down, in the skillet.
4. Quickly add your cheese slices on top of the bread in the skillet. If you want to include any additional ingredients like bacon, tomatoes, or onions, you can place them on top of the cheese.
5. Place the second slice of bread on top, buttered side up, to create a sandwich.
6. Cook the sandwich for a few minutes on each side, or until the bread is golden brown and crispy, and the cheese is melted. You can use a spatula to gently press down on the sandwich while cooking to help the cheese melt evenly.
7. Once the sandwich is cooked to your desired level of crispiness and the cheese is gooey, remove it from the skillet.
8. Let the sandwich cool for a minute or two to avoid burning your mouth, then cut it in half diagonally or into smaller portions if desired.
9. Serve your grilled cheese sandwich while it's still warm and enjoy!

Section 3

Snack Attack

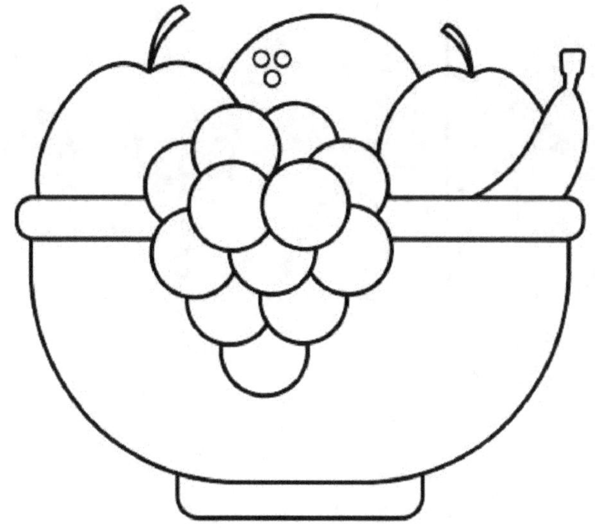

Ants on a log

Serves: 6   Prep time: 5 min   Cook time: 5min

INGREDIENTS

Celery sticks

(Peanut butter or an

alternative like almond

butter or cream cheese)

Raisins or other small dried

fruits (these are the "ants")

DIRECTIONS

1. Wash and cut the celery stalks into manageable lengths, usually about 3-4 inches long.
2. Spread a layer of peanut butter (or your preferred alternative) inside the concave side of each celery stick.
3. Place raisins or small dried fruits on top of the peanut butter. These represent the "ants" on the log.

Fruit Kabobs

INGREDIENTS

Assorted fruits (such as strawberries, pineapple chunks, melon balls, grapes, kiwi slices, and banana slices)

Wooden or metal skewers

DIRECTIONS

1. Wash and prepare the fruits by cutting them into bite-sized pieces or shapes that are suitable for skewering.
2. If you're using wooden skewers, soak them in water for about 30 minutes before assembling the kabobs. This helps prevent the skewers from burning during grilling or broiling.
3. Start assembling the fruit kabobs by sliding the prepared fruit pieces onto the skewers. You can arrange them in any pattern or order you prefer, making them as colorful and appealing as you like.
4. Place the assembled fruit kabobs on a platter or baking sheet. If you'd like, you can drizzle them with honey or sprinkle with a bit of lime or lemon juice for added flavor.
5. Fruit kabobs can be enjoyed as is, or you can grill them on a barbecue or broil them in the oven for a few minutes until the fruit begins to caramelize and develop grill marks. Be sure to monitor them closely to avoid overcooking.
6. Serve the fruit kabobs as a refreshing and healthy snack, dessert, or appetizer at parties and gatherings.

Popcorn Party

Serves: 6   Prep time: 3 min   Cook time: 5 min

INGREDIENTS

Offer a variety of popcorn flavors. You can have classic buttered popcorn, caramel popcorn, cheese popcorn, or even spicy popcorn. Consider making different batches or purchasing flavored popcorn

DIRECTIONS

1. Popcorn Varieties: Offer a variety of popcorn flavors. You can have classic buttered popcorn, caramel popcorn, cheese popcorn, or even spicy popcorn. Consider making different batches or purchasing flavored popcorn.

2. Popcorn Bar: Set up a popcorn bar with various toppings and seasonings. Include options like melted butter, chocolate drizzle, powdered seasonings (e.g., ranch, buffalo, barbecue), grated cheese, and mixed nuts.

3. Popcorn Seasonings: Provide a range of seasonings and spices for guests to customize their popcorn. Some popular options include nutritional yeast, cinnamon sugar, chili powder, and garlic salt.

4. Sweet Treats: Incorporate sweet treats alongside the savory popcorn options. You can have a candy station with chocolates, gummies, and other candies to mix into your popcorn.

Section 4

Dinnertime Adventures

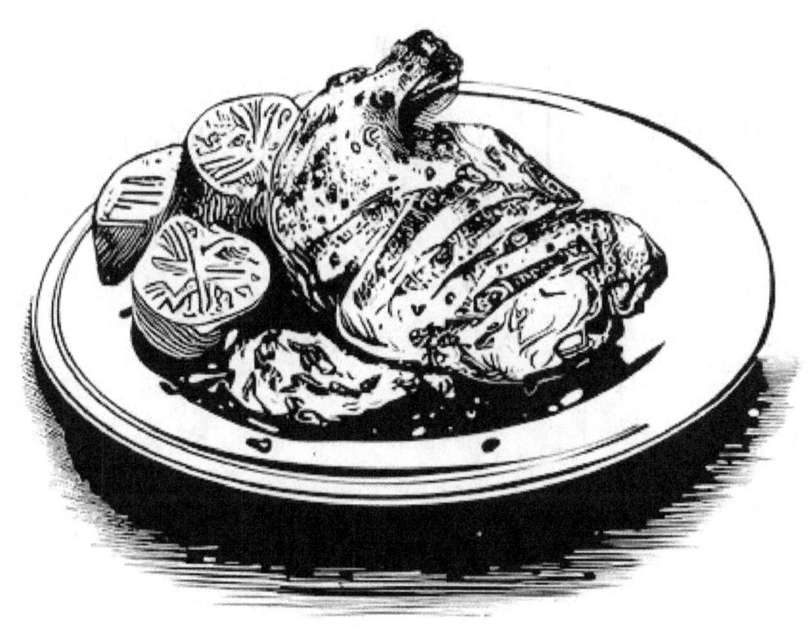

Spaghetti with Tomato Sauce

Serves: 6   Prep time: 10 min   Cook time: 30 min

INGREDIENTS

8 ounces of spaghetti

2 tablespoons olive oil

1 small onion, finely

chopped

2 cloves garlic, minced

1 (28-ounce) can of crushed

tomatoes

1 teaspoon dried basil

1 teaspoon dried oregano

Salt and pepper to taste

Pinch of red pepper flakes

(optional, for some heat)

Grated Parmesan cheese

(optional, for garnish)

Fresh basil leaves (optional,

for garnish)

DIRECTIONS

1. Cook the Spaghetti:
- Bring a large pot of salted water to a boil.
- Add the spaghetti and cook according to the package instructions until it's al dente, typically about 8-10 minutes.
- Drain the cooked spaghetti and set it aside.

2. Make the Tomato Sauce:
- In a large skillet or saucepan, heat the olive oil over medium heat.
- Add the chopped onion and cook for about 3-4 minutes until it becomes translucent.
- Stir in the minced garlic and cook for another 30 seconds until fragrant.
- Pour in the crushed tomatoes, dried basil, dried oregano, salt, pepper, and red pepper flakes (if using). Stir to combine.
- Bring the sauce to a simmer, then reduce the heat to low. Let it simmer for about 15-20 minutes, stirring occasionally, to allow the flavors to meld and the sauce to thicken slightly.

3. Combine and Serve:
- Once the tomato sauce is ready, add the cooked spaghetti to the skillet with the sauce.
- Toss the spaghetti in the sauce until it's well coated.
- Taste and adjust the seasoning with more salt, pepper, or red pepper flakes if needed.
- Serve the spaghetti with tomato sauce hot, garnished with grated Parmesan cheese and fresh basil leaves if desired.

Baked Chicken Tenders

Serves: 6   Prep time: 20 min   Cook time: 15 min

INGREDIENTS

1 pound chicken tenders or boneless, chicken breasts cut into strips

1 cup breadcrumbs (you can use panko breadcrumbs for extra crispiness)

1/2 cup grated Parmesan cheese (optional for added flavor)

1 teaspoon paprika

1/2 teaspoon garlic powder

1/2 teaspoon onion powder

1/2 teaspoon dried oregano or thyme

Salt and pepper to taste

2 large eggs, beaten

Cooking spray or a drizzle of olive oil

DIRECTIONS

1. Preheat your oven to 400°F (200°C) and line a baking sheet with parchment paper or lightly grease it with cooking spray.

2. In a shallow dish, combine the breadcrumbs, grated Parmesan cheese (if using), paprika, garlic powder, onion powder, dried oregano or thyme, salt, and pepper. Mix everything well to create your breading mixture.

3. In another shallow dish, beat the eggs.

4. Dip each chicken tender into the beaten eggs to coat it, then roll it in the breadcrumb mixture, pressing the breadcrumbs onto the chicken to ensure they adhere well.

5. Place the coated chicken tenders on the prepared baking sheet, leaving a little space between each piece.

6. If you want extra crispiness, you can lightly spray the tops of the chicken tenders with cooking spray or drizzle them with a bit of olive oil.

7. Bake in the preheated oven for about 15-20 minutes, or until the chicken is cooked through and the coating is golden brown and crispy. The exact cooking time may vary depending on the thickness of your chicken tenders, so use a meat thermometer to ensure the internal temperature reaches 165°F (74°C).

8. Once done, remove the baked chicken tenders from the oven and let them cool for a few minutes before serving.

Chicken Wraps

Serves: 4   Prep time: 21 min   Cook time: 6 min

INGREDIENTS

For the Chicken:

2 boneless, chicken breasts

1 tablespoon olive oil

1 teaspoon paprika

1/2 teaspoon garlic powder

Salt and pepper to taste

For the Wrap Assembly:

4 large tortillas or flatbreads

1 cup shredded lettuce

1 cup diced tomatoes

1/2 cup diced red onion

1/2 cup diced bell peppers (red, green, or yellow)

1/2 cup shredded cheddar cheese (or your preferred cheese)

1/4 cup sour cream or Greek yogurt

Salsa or hot sauce (optional for added flavor)

Sliced avocado or guacamole (optional)

DIRECTIONS

1. Prepare the Chicken:

- Season the chicken breasts with paprika, garlic powder, salt, and pepper.
- Heat the olive oil in a skillet over medium-high heat.
- Add the chicken breasts and cook for 6-8 minutes on each side or until they are cooked through and no longer pink in the center.
- Remove the chicken from the skillet and let it rest for a few minutes before slicing it into thin strips.

2. Assemble the Wraps:

- Lay out the tortillas or flatbreads on a clean surface.
- Place a layer of shredded lettuce down the center of each tortilla.
- Add the sliced chicken on top of the lettuce.

3. Add Vegetables and Condiments:

- Sprinkle diced tomatoes, red onion, and bell peppers over the chicken.
- Drizzle sour cream or Greek yogurt over the top for added creaminess.
- If desired, add salsa or hot sauce for extra flavor and heat.

4. Fold and Serve:

- Carefully fold in the sides of the tortilla and then roll it up from the bottom, creating a tight wrap.
- Repeat the process for the remaining tortillas.
- Serve the chicken wraps immediately, either whole or sliced in half diagonally for easy handling.

Section 5

Sweet Treats

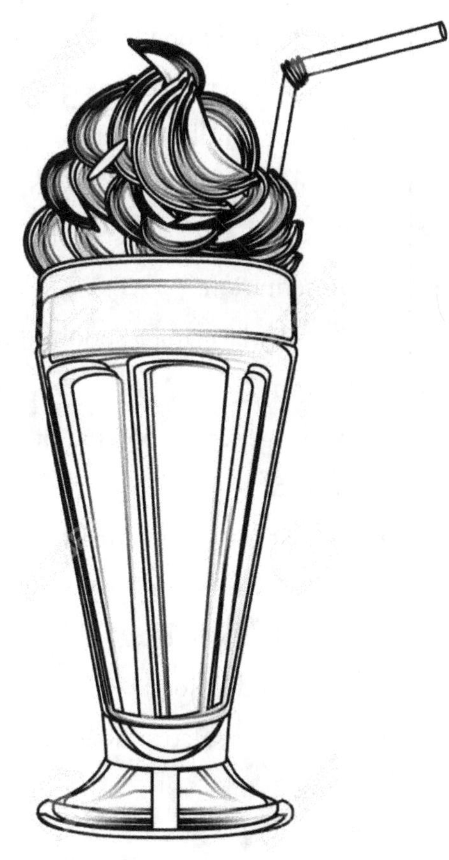

Fruit Salad Sundae

Serves: 4   Prep time: 20 min   Cook time: 45 min

INGREDIENTS

For the Fruit Salad:

Assorted fresh fruits (e.g., strawberries, blueberries, pineapple, grapes, kiwi, banana, etc.)

Fresh mint leaves (for garnish, optional)

For the Yogurt Topping:

Greek yogurt or your favorite yogurt

Honey or maple syrup (for sweetening, optional)

DIRECTIONS

1. Prepare the Fruits:
- Wash and peel (if necessary) the fruits.
- Cut them into bite-sized pieces. Try to keep the pieces relatively uniform in size for a visually appealing salad.
2. Mix the Fruit Salad:
- In a large bowl, combine the assorted fresh fruits.
- Gently toss them together to ensure an even distribution of flavors.
3. Prepare the Yogurt Topping:
- In a separate bowl, mix the Greek yogurt with a bit of honey or maple syrup for sweetness, if desired. You can also add a drop of vanilla extract for extra flavor.
- Assemble the Fruit Salad Sundae:
- To serve, you can use a clear glass or bowl for an attractive presentation.
- Start by layering a spoonful of the yogurt mixture at the bottom.
- Add a generous portion of the mixed fruit salad on top of the yogurt.
- Repeat the layers until you reach the top of the glass or bowl.
4. Finish with a dollop of yogurt and a sprig of fresh mint for garnish, if you like.
5. Serve and Enjoy:
- Your fruit salad sundae is ready to be enjoyed. Grab a spoon and dig in!

Strawberry Milkshake

Serves: 2   Prep time: 5 min   Cook time: 5 min

INGREDIENTS

1 cup strawberries

1 cup milk

2-4 tablespoons granulated

sugar

2-3 scoops of vanilla ice cream

Ice cubes (optional, for a

colder and thicker shake)

DIRECTIONS

1. Start by washing and hulling the strawberries. If you're using frozen strawberries, you can skip this step.
2. Place the strawberries in a blender.
3. Add the milk to the blender.
4. If you want your milkshake to be sweeter, add sugar to taste. Start with 2 tablespoons, blend, and taste. Add more sugar if needed.
5. If you want an extra creamy and sweet milkshake, add 2-3 scoops of vanilla ice cream to the blender. This step is optional but highly recommended for a classic milkshake flavor.
6. If you prefer a thicker milkshake or want to make it colder, you can add a few ice cubes to the blender.
7. Blend all the ingredients until smooth and well combined. If the milkshake is too thick, you can add more milk to reach your desired consistency.
8. Taste the milkshake and adjust the sweetness or thickness if necessary.
9. Once you're satisfied with the taste and texture, pour the strawberry milkshake into a glass.
10. Optionally, you can top the milkshake with whipped cream and garnish it with a fresh strawberry or a sprinkle of crushed graham crackers, chocolate shavings, or sprinkles for extra flair.
11. Serve the strawberry milkshake immediately with a straw and enjoy!

Rice Krispie Treat

Serves: 12   Prep time: 10 min   Cook time: 30 min

INGREDIENTS

6 cups of Rice Krispies cereal

1/4 cup (4 tablespoons) of unsalted

butter

1 package (10 ounces) of

marshmallows

DIRECTIONS

1. In a large saucepan, melt the butter over low heat.
2. Add the marshmallows to the melted butter and stir continuously until the marshmallows are completely melted and the mixture is smooth. This usually takes a few minutes.
3. Remove the saucepan from the heat and immediately add the Rice Krispies cereal. Stir quickly and thoroughly to coat the cereal evenly with the marshmallow mixture.
4. Once the cereal is well coated, transfer the mixture to a greased 9x13-inch (23x33 cm) baking pan or a similar-sized dish.
5. Use a greased spatula or your hands (make sure they are clean and greased) to press the mixture firmly into the pan. You want to make sure it's evenly spread and compacted.
6. Allow the Rice Krispie Treats to cool and set for at least 30 minutes. Once they've cooled and solidified, you can cut them into squares or rectangles.
7. Serve and enjoy!

Conclusion

"I hope you have as much fun making these recipes as you will eating them! Remember, cooking is a great way to learn new skills and spend time together as a family. So, keep experimenting in the kitchen, and who knows, maybe you'll become a famous chef one day. Happy cooking!"

Feel free to add colorful illustrations and photos to make the cookbook more engaging for children. Additionally, consider involving kids in the recipe testing and cooking process to make it a truly interactive and educational experience.

Your feedback is greatly appreciated!

It's through your feedback, support and reviews that I'm able to create the best books possible and serve more people.

I would be extremely grateful if you could take just 60 seconds to kindly leave an honest review of the book on Amazon. Please share your feedback and thoughts for others to see.

To do so, simply find the book on Amazon's website (or wherever you purchased the book from) and locate the section to leave a review. Select a star rating and write a couple of sentences.

That's it! Thank you so much for your support.

Review this product

Share your thoughts with other customers

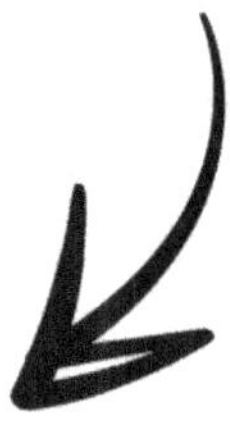

Write a customer review

References

OpenAI. (2023). Conversations with ChatGPT. Retrieved [insert date], from https://www.openai.com/chatgpt/

www.ingramcontent.com/pod-product-compliance
Lightning Source LLC
Chambersburg PA
CBHW080734260726
48660CB00010B/3847